CONQUERING TINEA VERSICOLOR

A Complete Guide to Skin Health and Nourishing Food Recipes to Combat Fungal Infections

Dr. Oftelith S.

Copyright©2024 Dr. Oftelith S.

All rights reserved.

Disclaimer

The information provided in this book is intended for personal and educational purposes only. It is not a substitute for professional medical advice, diagnosis, or treatment. Readers are urged to consult healthcare professionals for personalized guidance. The author and publisher disclaim any responsibility for adverse effects resulting from the information. Individuals diagnosed with one problem or another are advised to undergo regular medical check-ups and consult with healthcare experts for ongoing monitoring and necessary advice. The contents of this book are not for sale or public use without explicit permission, emphasizing the importance of respecting intellectual property rights.

Table of Contents

Introduction 4
Brief History 7
Clear Definition 10
Symptoms of Tinea Versicolor 11
Causes of Tinea Versicolor 14
Areas Affected by Tinea Versicolor 19
    Tinea Versicolor on the Face 20
    Tinea Versicolor and Vitiligo 20
    Tinea Versicolor and Pityriasis Rosea 22
Diagnosis of Tinea Versicolor 25
Treatment of Tinea Versicolor 27
Conclusion 33
Appendix 35
    Medical Tips and Advice 35
    Facts About Tinea Versicolor 40
25 Food Recipes 44
Glossary of Terms 69

Introduction

Do you know that being careless with your skin can cause you significant issues later on? It's easy to focus on internal health and forget about the skin, which is our largest organ and the first line of defense against the outside world. One of the problems that can afflict your skin is called Tinea Versicolor. Have you heard of it before? Let me assume 80% of people haven't. Tinea Versicolor is a fungal infection that results in patches of discolored spots on your skin.

I'm sure you're not entirely clear about it yet, but as we delve deeper, you'll understand everything you need to know about Tinea Versicolor. As a health researcher, I always encourage everyone to pay attention to their health, both inwardly and outwardly. You shouldn't focus solely on one aspect of your health; remember, when you're healthy, that's when you can think about achievements and manage your daily activities effectively.

This particular skin problem causes a lot of discomfort, especially during hotter weather, and can be quite painful. It's not something to overlook. Come closer, and let's educate ourselves, as this knowledge will help you and others.

You don't need to wait until you're diagnosed to learn about this condition. Knowledge is valuable and should be acquired daily. Are you ready to learn? Jump right in and don't miss any part of this manual.

Brief History

Tinea versicolor, also known as pityriasis versicolor, has been recognized for centuries as a distinct dermatological condition. The term "tinea" historically referred to fungal infections of the skin, while "versicolor" indicates the variable coloration of the skin affected by the condition.

The condition was first described in the early 19th century, and its fungal origin was identified in the late 19th and early 20th centuries. It became clear that the causative agents were species of Malassezia, a genus of yeast that is part of the normal flora of human skin.

Initially, Malassezia furfur was considered the primary culprit. However, further research in the latter half of the 20th century identified Malassezia globosa as the most common species responsible for Tinea versicolor, with Malassezia furfur contributing to a smaller percentage of cases.

The condition has been documented worldwide, but it is particularly prevalent in tropical and subtropical regions, where warm and humid climates promote the overgrowth of Malassezia yeasts. These yeasts thrive in environments rich in skin oils (lipids) and dead skin cells, which explains the higher incidence of Tinea versicolor among adolescents and young adults who tend to have oilier skin.

Throughout history, treatments have evolved from traditional remedies to modern antifungal medications. Early treatments included sulfur and tar preparations, which were later replaced by more effective topical and systemic antifungal agents such as ketoconazole, selenium sulfide, and itraconazole.

Despite its long history, Tinea versicolor remains a common and sometimes recurrent condition, emphasizing the need for ongoing education and effective management strategies. Advances in dermatological research continue to improve our understanding and treatment of this persistent skin infection.

Clear Definition

Tinea versicolor is a frequently occurring fungal skin infection. This condition arises when the fungus disrupts the skin's normal pigmentation, leading to the appearance of small, discolored spots. These spots can be either lighter or darker than the surrounding skin and typically appear on the trunk and shoulders.

Symptoms of Tinea Versicolor

Tinea versicolor is an infection that attacks the skin and can manifest in several distinctive ways, depending on the case.

- **Discolored Patches**: One of the most noticeable signs is the presence of patches on the skin that are either lighter or darker than the surrounding area. These patches can vary in color, appearing white, pink, red, or brown.

- **Location**: The discolored spots are most commonly found on the trunk, such as the chest and back, as well as the shoulders and upper arms. Occasionally, they may also appear on the neck.

- **Texture**: The affected areas often have a dry and scaly texture. When touched, the skin in these patches may feel rougher than the surrounding healthy skin.

- **Visibility Changes**: These spots can become more apparent when the skin is exposed to sunlight. The patches do not tan like the rest of the skin, making them stand out more during the summer or in sunny climates.

- **Itching or Discomfort**: Although not always present, some individuals may experience mild itching or discomfort in the areas affected by Tinea versicolor. However, these symptoms are generally rare and not severe.

- **Weather Impact**: The condition tends to worsen in warm and humid weather, which can cause the patches to become more pronounced. Conversely, the symptoms may improve or become less noticeable during cooler weather.

- **Chronic and Recurrent Nature**: Tinea versicolor can be a chronic condition, with symptoms that may recur, especially if the individual lives in a hot, humid environment or has naturally oily skin.

Causes of Tinea Versicolor

Tinea versicolor is caused by the overgrowth of a type of yeast known as Malassezia, which is naturally found on the skin. Several factors can contribute to this overgrowth, leading to the development of the infection.

- **Natural Skin Flora**: Malassezia yeast normally resides on healthy skin without causing any issues. It thrives on the natural oils (lipids) and dead skin cells present on the skin's surface.

- **Warm and Humid Environments**: The condition is more common in hot and humid climates. These environmental factors create an ideal breeding ground for the yeast, promoting its excessive growth.

➤ **Oily Skin**: Individuals with naturally oily skin are more susceptible to Tinea versicolor. The excess oil provides additional nutrients that the yeast needs to multiply.

➤ **Sweating**: Excessive sweating can also contribute to the overgrowth of Malassezia yeast. Sweat increases moisture on the skin, further supporting the yeast's proliferation.

➤ **Hormonal Changes**: Hormonal fluctuations, particularly those that increase oil production in the skin, can trigger the onset of Tinea versicolor. This is why the condition is often observed in adolescents and young adults who are undergoing hormonal changes.

- **Weakened Immune System**: A compromised immune system can make it difficult for the body to keep the yeast population under control, leading to overgrowth and infection. This can occur in individuals with conditions such as diabetes or those taking immunosuppressive medications.

- **Associated Skin Conditions**: People with certain skin conditions like seborrheic dermatitis, dandruff, and hyperhidrosis (excessive sweating) are at higher risk of developing Tinea versicolor. These conditions create an environment that is conducive to the yeast's growth.

- **Non-Contagious Nature**: Despite being an infection, Tinea versicolor is not contagious. The yeast responsible for the condition is already present on the skin of most individuals, and the infection occurs due to the factors mentioned above rather than through direct transmission from person to person.

Note

This skin disease frequently affects adolescents and young adults, particularly in warm and humid climates. The yeast responsible for the infection thrives on skin oils (lipids) and dead skin cells.

People with seborrheic dermatitis, dandruff, and hyperhidrosis are more prone to developing this condition.

Areas Affected by Tinea Versicolor

Tinea versicolor primarily occurs on the upper body, including:

- **Trunk**: The chest and back are the most common areas where discolored patches appear.

- **Shoulders**: The infection often extends to the shoulders, particularly in individuals who sweat excessively.

- **Neck**: Patches can also manifest on the neck, where oil and sweat accumulation is common.

- **Upper Arms**: The upper arms are frequently affected, especially in warm and humid environments.

Tinea Versicolor on the Face

While Tinea versicolor can occasionally appear on the face, it is less common. Facial involvement might lead to confusion with other skin conditions. The discolored spots on the face may be more prominent due to increased visibility and can sometimes be mistaken for other dermatological issues.

Tinea Versicolor and Vitiligo

➢ **Tinea Versicolor**

- **Cause**: Fungal infection caused by Malassezia yeast.

- **Symptoms**: Discolored patches that can be white, pink, red, or brown, with a scaly texture.

- **Location**: Typically affects the trunk, shoulders, neck, and upper arms.

- **Other Characteristics**: May cause mild itching and tends to worsen in warm, humid conditions.

➢ **Vitiligo**

- **Cause**: Autoimmune condition where the immune system attacks melanocytes, the cells responsible for producing skin pigment.

- **Symptoms**: Smooth, white patches on the skin that lack pigment.

- **Location**: Can occur anywhere on the body, often around the mouth, eyes, and on the hands and feet.

- **Other Characteristics**: Does not cause itching or discomfort and is more noticeable on darker skin.

Tinea Versicolor and Pityriasis Rosea
> **Tinea Versicolor**

- **Cause**: Overgrowth of Malassezia yeast.

- **Symptoms**: Small, discolored patches that may be scaly and mildly itchy.

- **Location**: Mostly affects the trunk and shoulders.

- **Other Characteristics**: Chronic and recurrent, especially in humid climates.

➢ **Pityriasis Rosea**

- **Cause**: Believed to be associated with viral infections, particularly certain herpes viruses.

- **Symptoms**: Starts with a large, single patch (herald patch) followed by smaller lesions. The rash often forms a "Christmas tree" pattern on the back.

- **Location**: Commonly appears on the chest, abdomen, and back.

- **Other Characteristics**: Can be mildly itchy and usually resolves on its own within 6-8 weeks.

Diagnosis of Tinea Versicolor

Diagnosing Tinea versicolor generally involves a visual inspection by a healthcare professional to identify the typical features of the rash. Several additional diagnostic methods can be used to confirm the presence of the infection:

➢ **Visual Examination**

A doctor will look at the affected skin to identify the distinctive discolored patches, which can range in color and are often slightly scaly.

➢ **Wood's Lamp**

Using ultraviolet light, a doctor can examine the skin. Affected areas may glow with a yellow-green or coppery-orange hue, which helps in distinguishing Tinea versicolor from other conditions.

➢ Microscopic Analysis

Skin cells scraped from the affected area can be treated with potassium hydroxide (KOH) and examined under a microscope. This method reveals the yeast cells in a characteristic pattern resembling "spaghetti and meatballs," which is indicative of Tinea versicolor.

➢ Skin Biopsy

In some instances, a small piece of skin may be removed for a thorough examination. This helps to exclude other skin disorders that might resemble Tinea versicolor.

Treatment of Tinea Versicolor

Managing Tinea versicolor involves a combination of topical and oral antifungal medications, lifestyle adjustments, and preventive measures to effectively eliminate the infection and reduce the likelihood of recurrence.

➢ **Topical Antifungals**

- **Lotions, Creams, and Gels**: Medications such as clotrimazole, miconazole, and terbinafine can be directly applied to the affected skin. These treatments are generally used once or twice daily for about 2 to 4 weeks. They work by inhibiting the growth of the yeast responsible for the infection.

- **Shampoos and Foams**: Products containing selenium sulfide, ketoconazole, or zinc pyrithione can be used on larger affected areas. These are often applied to the skin, left on for a specific duration (usually 10-15 minutes), and then rinsed off. Treatment duration may vary, but it typically lasts from several days to a couple of weeks.

➢ **Oral Antifungals**

- In cases where topical treatments are not effective or the infection is widespread, oral antifungal medications such as fluconazole or itraconazole may be prescribed. These medications are usually taken for a short duration, often a single dose or for several days. Oral antifungals can provide a more systemic approach to eliminating the yeast.

➢ **Preventive Measures**

- **Regular Use of Medicated Cleansers**: To prevent recurrence, individuals might use antifungal shampoos or body washes weekly or bi-weekly. Products containing selenium sulfide, ketoconazole, or zinc pyrithione are often recommended.

- **Maintaining Dry and Cool Skin**: Since the yeast thrives in warm and humid conditions, keeping the skin dry and cool can help prevent overgrowth. Wearing breathable fabrics like cotton and avoiding excessive sweating can be beneficial.

- **Avoiding Oily Skin Products**: Reducing the use of oily or greasy skin products can limit the nutrients available to the yeast, thereby controlling its growth.

➢ **Natural and Home Remedies**

- **Aloe Vera**: Known for its soothing properties, aloe vera gel can help relieve itching and irritation associated with Tinea versicolor. Some studies suggest it may also inhibit yeast growth.

- **Honey and Olive Oil**: A mixture of honey, olive oil, and beeswax has been found to have antifungal properties and can be applied to the affected areas.

- **Turmeric**: This spice, which has anti-inflammatory and antifungal properties, can be made into a paste and applied to the skin. Turmeric creams are also available commercially.

➢ **Long-term Management**

- For those prone to recurrent infections, long-term management strategies are essential. This may include the regular use of antifungal treatments, lifestyle changes to reduce moisture on the skin, and avoiding triggers such as excessive heat and humidity.

- **Sun Exposure**: Protecting the skin from excessive sun exposure by using broad-spectrum, non-greasy sunscreen with at least SPF 30 can prevent the patches from becoming more noticeable.

Conclusion

If you have truly read every page of this book, you now possess a comprehensive understanding of Tinea Versicolor, a fungal skin infection. Beyond simply familiarizing yourself with this condition, you have equipped yourself with in-depth knowledge about its causes, symptoms, and treatments, including effective home management strategies. This book has also provided you with valuable food recipes to support your skin's health and recovery.

With this newfound knowledge, you are well-prepared to recognize and address Tinea Versicolor. Do not allow your skin to suffer from infections; pay attention to its needs just as you do to other parts of your body. Your overall well-being is paramount, so take good care of yourself!

Appendix

Medical Tips and Advice

- **Early Diagnosis**: Seek medical advice as soon as you notice unusual patches on your skin for early diagnosis and treatment.

- **Use Antifungal Products**: Regularly use antifungal creams, lotions, or shampoos as prescribed by your doctor to manage and prevent the infection.

- **Maintain Dry Skin**: Keep your skin dry and cool, especially in humid environments, to prevent yeast overgrowth.

- **Avoid Oily Products**: Steer clear of oily skin products that can feed the yeast and exacerbate the condition.

- **Wear Breathable Fabrics**: Choose loose, breathable fabrics like cotton to reduce sweating and allow your skin to breathe.

- **Use Sunscreen**: Apply broad-spectrum, non-greasy sunscreen with at least SPF 30 to protect your skin and prevent the patches from becoming more noticeable.

- **Hygiene Practices**: Maintain good hygiene by showering regularly and thoroughly drying your skin afterward.

- **Avoid Excessive Sun Exposure**: Limit sun exposure, as tanning can make the discolored patches more visible.

- **Regular Check-ups**: Schedule regular check-ups with your healthcare provider to monitor and manage the condition effectively.

- **Natural Remedies**: Consider natural remedies like aloe vera, honey, and turmeric for additional relief, but use them as a supplement to medical treatments.

- **Stay Hydrated**: Embrace drinking plenty of water to keep your skin hydrated and healthy.

- **Balanced Diet**: Choose a balanced diet rich in vitamins and minerals to support overall skin health.

- **Manage Stress**: Reduce stress through relaxation techniques, as stress can weaken your immune system and exacerbate skin conditions.

- **Regular Exercise**: Engage in regular physical activity to boost your immune system, but make sure to shower and dry off afterward to prevent sweat buildup.

- **Avoid Sharing Personal Items**: Do not share towels, clothing, or personal care items to reduce the risk of spreading any skin-related infections.

- **Follow Treatment Plans**: Adhere to the full course of treatment prescribed by your doctor, even if symptoms improve, to ensure complete eradication of the infection.

- **Educate Yourself**: Stay informed about Tinea versicolor and its management to make proactive choices about your skin health.

Facts About Tinea Versicolor

- **Common Fungal Infection**: Tinea versicolor is a frequent skin condition caused by the overgrowth of yeast on the skin.

- **Discolored Patches**: It results in small, discolored patches that can be lighter or darker than the surrounding skin.

- **Areas Affected**: The condition typically affects the trunk, shoulders, and proximal extremities.

- **Causing Yeast**: The primary yeast responsible is Malassezia globosa, with Malassezia furfur causing fewer cases.

- **Environmental Triggers**: Warm and humid climates can trigger the overgrowth of the yeast, leading to infection.

- **Not Contagious**: Tinea versicolor is not contagious and cannot be spread from person to person.

- **Prevalent in Adolescents and Young Adults**: It commonly affects adolescents and young adults, particularly those with oily skin or living in humid environments.

- **Recurrence**: The condition can recur, especially in warm weather, requiring ongoing treatment and preventive measures.

- **Treatment**: Antifungal treatments, including topical creams, shampoos, and oral medications, are effective in managing the infection.

- **Diagnosis**: Diagnosis can be confirmed through visual examination, Wood's lamp, KOH test, or skin biopsy.

- **Healing Time**: Treatment clears the infection in about 2 to 4 weeks, but skin discoloration may take several months to a year to resolve.

- **Natural Remedies**: Aloe vera, honey, and turmeric are natural treatments that may help manage symptoms.

- **Preventive Measures**: Regular use of antifungal shampoos, maintaining dry skin, and avoiding oily skin products can help prevent recurrence.

- **Emotional Impact**: The condition can cause emotional distress and self-consciousness due to its visible nature.

- **Associated Conditions**: More common in individuals with seborrheic dermatitis, dandruff, and hyperhidrosis.

25 Food Recipes

➤ Turmeric Golden Milk

Ingredients

- *2 cups almond milk*
- *1 tsp turmeric powder*
- *1/2 tsp cinnamon powder*
- *1/4 tsp ginger powder*
- *1 tbsp honey*
- *Pinch of black pepper*

Preparation

1. Heat the almond milk in a saucepan over medium heat.
2. Add turmeric, cinnamon, ginger, and black pepper.

3. Stir well and let it simmer for 5 minutes.

4. Add honey before serving.

➢ Garlic and Spinach Soup

Ingredients

- *1 tbsp olive oil*
- *4 cloves garlic, minced*
- *1 onion, chopped*
- *4 cups spinach leaves*
- *4 cups vegetable broth*
- *Salt and pepper to taste*

Preparation

1. Heat olive oil in a pot and sauté garlic and onion until fragrant.

2. Add spinach and cook until wilted.

3. Pour in the vegetable broth, bring to a boil, then simmer for 15 minutes.
4. Season with salt and pepper.

➤ **Ginger Tea**

Ingredients

- *1 inch fresh ginger root, sliced*
- *2 cups water*
- *1 tbsp honey*
- *1 tbsp lemon juice*

Preparation

1. Boil water and add ginger slices.
2. Simmer for 10 minutes.
3. Strain the tea and add honey and lemon juice.

➢ Salmon with Avocado Salsa

Ingredients

- *2 salmon fillets*
- *1 tbsp olive oil*
- *Salt and pepper to taste*
- *1 avocado, diced*
- *1 tomato, diced*
- *1/4 cup red onion, chopped*
- *1 tbsp lime juice*
- *1 tbsp cilantro, chopped*

Preparation

1. Season salmon with salt and pepper, then grill or bake at 375°F for 15-20 minutes.

2. Mix avocado, tomato, red onion, lime juice, and cilantro in a bowl.

3. Serve salmon topped with avocado salsa.

➤ **Greek Yogurt with Honey and Nuts**

Ingredients

- *1 cup Greek yogurt*
- *1 tbsp honey*
- *2 tbsp mixed nuts*

Preparation

1. Scoop Greek yogurt into a bowl.
2. Drizzle with honey and sprinkle with mixed nuts.

➤ **Quinoa Salad with Lemon Vinaigrette**

Ingredients

- 1 cup quinoa
- 2 cups water
- 1 cucumber, diced
- 1 bell pepper, diced
- 1/4 cup red onion, chopped
- 1/4 cup feta cheese, crumbled
- 1/4 cup olive oil
- 2 tbsp lemon juice
- Salt and pepper to taste

Preparation

1. Cook quinoa in water according to package instructions and let cool.

2. Mix quinoa, cucumber, bell pepper, red onion, and feta in a large bowl.

3. In a small bowl, whisk olive oil, lemon juice, salt, and pepper.

4. Pour vinaigrette over salad and toss.

➢ Cucumber Mint Water

Ingredients

- *1 cucumber, sliced*
- *10 mint leaves*
- *2 liters water*

Preparation

1. Combine cucumber slices and mint leaves in a pitcher.

2. Fill with water and refrigerate for at least 2 hours before serving.

➤ Blueberry Almond Smoothie

Ingredients

- *1 cup blueberries*
- *1 banana*
- *1/2 cup almond milk*
- *1 tbsp almond butter*
- *1 tbsp honey*

Preparation

1. Blend all ingredients until smooth.
2. Pour into a glass and serve immediately.

➤ Turmeric Rice

Ingredients

- *1 cup basmati rice*
- *2 cups water*
- *1 tsp turmeric powder*
- *1 tbsp olive oil*
- *Salt to taste*

Preparation

1. Rinse rice under cold water.
2. In a pot, heat olive oil and add turmeric powder.
3. Add rice and water, then bring to a boil.
4. Reduce heat, cover, and simmer until water is absorbed and rice is tender.

➢ **Avocado and Tomato Toast**

Ingredients

- *2 slices whole grain bread*
- *1 avocado, mashed*
- *1 tomato, sliced*
- *Salt and pepper to taste*

Preparation

1. Toast the bread.
2. Spread mashed avocado on each slice.
3. Top with tomato slices and season with salt and pepper.

➢ **Green Smoothie**

Ingredients

- *1 cup spinach*

- 1/2 cup kale
- 1 banana
- 1 apple, cored and chopped
- 1/2 cup water or coconut water

Preparation

1. Blend all ingredients until smooth.
2. Serve immediately.

➤ **Mango Chia Pudding**

Ingredients

- 1 cup coconut milk
- 1/2 cup chia seeds
- 1 mango, pureed
- 1 tbsp honey

Preparation

1. Mix coconut milk, chia seeds, and honey in a bowl.
2. Let it sit in the fridge for at least 2 hours or overnight.
3. Top with mango puree before serving.

➢ **Roasted Beet Salad**

Ingredients

- *4 beets, roasted and sliced*
- *1/4 cup goat cheese, crumbled*
- *1/4 cup walnuts, toasted*
- *2 tbsp olive oil*
- *1 tbsp balsamic vinegar*
- *Salt and pepper to taste*

Preparation

1. Toss roasted beets, goat cheese, and walnuts in a bowl.
2. Whisk olive oil, balsamic vinegar, salt, and pepper in a small bowl.
3. Pour dressing over salad and mix well.

➤ **Garlic Roasted Broccoli**

Ingredients

- *1 head broccoli, cut into florets*
- *3 cloves garlic, minced*
- *2 tbsp olive oil*
- *Salt and pepper to taste*

Preparation

1. Preheat oven to 400°F.
2. Toss broccoli with garlic, olive oil, salt, and pepper.
3. Spread on a baking sheet and roast for 20-25 minutes.

➢ **Carrot Ginger Soup**

Ingredients

- *1 tbsp olive oil*
- *1 onion, chopped*
- *2 cloves garlic, minced*
- *5 carrots, chopped*
- *1 inch ginger root, grated*
- *4 cups vegetable broth*
- *Salt and pepper to taste*

Preparation

1. Heat olive oil in a pot and sauté onion and garlic until fragrant.
2. Add carrots and ginger, and cook for 5 minutes.
3. Pour in vegetable broth, bring to a boil, then simmer until carrots are tender.
4. Blend until smooth and season with salt and pepper.

➢ **Berry and Spinach Salad**

Ingredients

- *2 cups spinach*
- *1 cup mixed berries (strawberries, blueberries, raspberries)*

- 1/4 cup almonds, sliced
- 1/4 cup feta cheese, crumbled
- 2 tbsp olive oil
- 1 tbsp balsamic vinegar

Preparation

1. Combine spinach, berries, almonds, and feta in a bowl.
2. Whisk olive oil and balsamic vinegar together and drizzle over salad.

➤ **Cinnamon Apple Oatmeal**

Ingredients

- 1 cup rolled oats
- 2 cups water or milk
- 1 apple, chopped

- *1 tsp cinnamon*
- *1 tbsp honey*

Preparation

1. Cook oats in water or milk according to package instructions.
2. Stir in chopped apple, cinnamon, and honey.
3. Serve warm.

➢ **Coconut Chia Smoothie Bowl**

Ingredients

- *1 cup coconut milk*
- *1/4 cup chia seeds*
- *1 banana, sliced*
- *1/2 cup berries*

- *1 tbsp shredded coconut*

Preparation

1. Mix coconut milk and chia seeds and refrigerate overnight.
2. Pour chia mixture into a bowl and top with banana, berries, and shredded coconut.

➢ Lemon Ginger Detox Drink

Ingredients

- *1 lemon, juiced*
- *1 inch ginger root, grated*
- *2 cups water*
- *1 tbsp honey*

Preparation

1. Mix lemon juice, grated ginger, and water.
2. Add honey and stir well.

➤ Tomato Basil Soup

Ingredients

- *1 tbsp olive oil*
- *1 onion, chopped*
- *3 cloves garlic, minced*
- *6 tomatoes, chopped*
- *2 cups vegetable broth*
- *1/4 cup fresh basil, chopped*
- *Salt and pepper to taste*

Preparation

1. Heat olive oil in a pot and sauté onion and garlic until fragrant.

2. Add tomatoes and cook for 10 minutes.

3. Pour in vegetable broth and bring to a boil, then simmer for 20 minutes.

4. Blend until smooth and stir in basil. Season with salt and pepper.

➢ **Quinoa Stuffed Peppers**

Ingredients

- 4 bell peppers, halved and seeded
- 1 cup cooked quinoa
- 1 can black beans, drained and rinsed
- 1 cup corn kernels
- 1/2 cup salsa
- 1/4 cup cilantro, chopped

Preparation

1. Preheat oven to 375°F.
2. Mix quinoa, black beans, corn, salsa, and cilantro in a bowl.
3. Stuff bell peppers with quinoa mixture.
4. Bake for 25-30 minutes.

➢ Avocado and Chickpea Salad

Ingredients

- *1 can chickpeas, drained and rinsed*
- *1 avocado, diced*
- *1 tomato, chopped*
- *1/4 cup red onion, chopped*
- *2 tbsp olive oil*
- *1 tbsp lemon juice*
- *Salt and pepper to taste*

Preparation

1. Mix chickpeas, avocado, tomato, and red onion in a bowl.
2. Whisk olive oil, lemon juice, salt, and pepper in a small bowl.
3. Pour dressing over salad and toss.

➢ **Spiced Lentil Soup**

Ingredients

- *1 tbsp olive oil*
- *1 onion, chopped*
- *3 cloves garlic, minced*
- *1 cup lentils, rinsed*
- *4 cups vegetable broth*
- *1 tsp cumin*

- *1/2 tsp turmeric*
- *1/4 tsp cayenne pepper*
- *Salt and pepper to taste*

Preparation

1. Heat olive oil in a pot and sauté onion and garlic until fragrant.
2. Add lentils, vegetable broth, cumin, turmeric, and cayenne pepper.
3. Bring to a boil, then simmer until lentils are tender. Season with salt and pepper.

➢ **Turmeric Cauliflower Rice**

Ingredients

- 1 head cauliflower, grated
- 1 tbsp olive oil

- 1 tsp turmeric powder
- Salt and pepper to taste

Preparation

1. Heat olive oil in a pan and add grated cauliflower.
2. Stir in turmeric and cook until cauliflower is tender.

➤ **Berry Kefir Smoothie**

Ingredients

- 1 cup kefir
- 1/2 cup mixed berries
- 1 banana
- 1 tbsp honey

Preparation

1. Blend all ingredients until smooth.

2. Serve immediately.

Glossary of Terms

Antifungal: Medications used to treat fungal infections by killing or stopping the growth of fungi. These can be topical (applied to the skin) or oral (taken by mouth).

Biopsy: A medical procedure in which a small sample of skin or other tissue is taken for examination under a microscope to diagnose a condition.

Clotrimazole: An antifungal medication commonly used to treat skin infections such as athlete's foot, jock itch, and Tinea Versicolor.

Discoloration: A change in the natural color of the skin, often seen as patches that are lighter or darker than the surrounding skin.

Fluconazole: An oral antifungal medication used to treat serious fungal infections, including Tinea Versicolor.

Hyphae: The long, branching structures of a fungus that are seen under a microscope and are part of the characteristic "spaghetti and meatballs" appearance in Tinea Versicolor.

Itraconazole: An oral antifungal drug used to treat a variety of fungal infections, including Tinea Versicolor.

Ketoconazole: An antifungal medication available in both topical and oral forms, used to treat fungal infections of the skin and other areas.

Malassezia: A genus of yeast that lives on the skin and can cause Tinea Versicolor when it overgrows.

Microscopy: The use of a microscope to examine small samples, such as skin cells, to diagnose conditions like Tinea Versicolor.

Pigmentation: The natural color of the skin, which can be affected by infections, leading to discoloration.

Potassium Hydroxide (KOH) Test: A diagnostic test where skin scrapings are treated with potassium hydroxide and examined under a microscope to detect fungal infections.

Recurrence: The return of an infection after it has been treated and initially cleared.

Selenium Sulfide: An antifungal agent found in shampoos and lotions used to treat Tinea Versicolor and dandruff.

Seborrheic Dermatitis: A common skin condition causing scaly, itchy patches, often affecting oily areas like the scalp, face, and upper body.

Selsun Blue: A brand of dandruff shampoo containing selenium sulfide, also used to treat Tinea Versicolor.

Topical: Medications or treatments applied directly to the skin rather than taken orally or injected.

Turmeric: A spice with anti-inflammatory and antifungal properties, sometimes used in natural remedies for skin conditions.

Ultraviolet (UV) Light: Light used in diagnostic tools like the Wood's lamp to help detect certain skin conditions, including Tinea Versicolor.

Vitiligo: A condition in which the immune system attacks pigment-producing cells in the skin, causing white patches that are smooth and not scaly.

Wood's Lamp: A diagnostic tool that emits ultraviolet light to examine the skin. It can highlight areas affected by fungal infections like Tinea Versicolor by causing them to fluoresce.

www.ingramcontent.com/pod-product-compliance
Lightning Source LLC
Chambersburg PA
CBHW070123230526
45472CB00004B/1394